My Gluten-Free Knoxville
a gluten-free-friendly all-American town

Your gluten-free guide to area markets, restaurants,
and lifestyle information.
Including online sources and apps for finding gluten-free restaurants

With excerpts from *Gluten-Free Mainstream America* on coping with celiac disease and gluten intolerance, and a national resource guide for gluten-free information.

by
Janet McKenzie Prince

My Gluten-Free Knoxville
Copyright © 2013 Janet McKenzie Prince
All rights reserved

ISBN 978-0-9667286-9-9 Revised Edition July 2013
Original Edition 2008 ISBN 978-0-9667286-4-4

Printed and published in the United States of America

No part of this book may be used or reproduced in any manner whatsoever without written permission of the author, except in the case of brief quotations embodied in critical articles and reviews.

White Dog Studio Productions
PO Box 198
Louisville, Tennessee 37777

www.missjanetsglutenfreeamerica.com

Book design and cover design by Janet McKenzie Prince

Although the author and publisher have exhaustively researched many sources to ensure the accuracy and completeness of the information in this book, we assume no responsibility for errors, inaccuracies, omissions, or any inconsistency herein. No information contained herein should be construed as medical advice or as a guarantee that individuals will tolerate foods prepared from these recipes.

My Gluten-Free Knoxville News Update

Since I first introduced *My Gluten-Free Knoxville* in 2008, and its revised editions thereafter, it has been a staple resource guide for our gluten-free community in the Knoxville area. I'm pleased to report that since the first edition, our local gluten-free sources have increased by leaps and bounds. Most of our local markets not only carry gluten-free products, but they offer us a wide variety of safe products from which to choose. Many local restaurants and fast-food establishments offer gluten-free menus. Our medical community provides us with professional and caring guidance. And an increasing number of local registered dietitians understand our dietary requirements. All of these advances are extremely important to us in the gluten-free community.

Remember, the only treatment for celiac disease is a strict adherence to a gluten-free diet. Eliminating gluten and eating nutritional, safe food is our direct path to good health. All of us who fall under the umbrella of gluten intolerance, including celiac disease, wheat allergies, and non-celiac gluten sensitivity, benefit from the wholesome support we receive within our gluten-free-friendly all-American town of Knoxville, Tennessee.

I said it before, and it's worth repeating: Knoxville is a wonderful place to live gluten free. We have our community's understanding and support. Therefore, the entire community benefits, because all its citizens have the opportunity to be healthy and productive.

Because of the positive changes in gluten-free awareness over the years, I've written more books to disseminate updated and additional information, not only to our local community, but to a national audience, as well. Gluten free has gone mainstream, and Knoxville, Tennessee is one of the leaders in the gluten-free revolution that has swept across our nation.

Here is a listing of my new series of books offered under the umbrella of Miss Janet's Gluten-Free America. (www.missjanetsglutenfreeamerica)

My Gluten-Free Knoxville is specific to the gluten-free friendly all-American town of Knoxville, Tennessee. It tells you where to shop, where to eat, who to talk to. This is your gluten-free guide to area markets, restaurants, and life-style information. Also included in the Knoxville guide are excerpts on coping with gluten intolerance from *Gluten-Free Mainstream America*.

Gluten-Free Mainstream America: Recipes for Health, featuring artisan breads, nutritional meals, how-to-instructions for coping with the cooking for celiac disease and gluten intolerance. The cookbook and guide includes my new book, *Miss Janet's American Breadbasket, Artisan Gluten-Free Breads and Baked Goods* in its entirety.

Miss Janet's American Breadbasket, Artisan Gluten-Free Breads and Baked Goods is also available under separate cover. For those who wish only the baking recipes, this book does not contain meal recipes, coping advice, nor the in-depth national resource guides included in *Gluten-Free Mainstream America.*

And simply for the love of good food and good health, ***New Cooks in America, Learning to Cook for a Healthier America,*** not only teaches you how to cook, but it shows you "How to Set Up your New Kitchen and How to Survive in It." Whether you are a young professional, a school kid starting out on your own, a couple of newlyweds setting up your first kitchen, or newly single and starting over, *New Cooks in America* will guide you gently through a delightful wholesome adventure inside your own kitchen.

These books are available on Amazon through my websites:
missjanetsglutenfreeamerica.com
and
newcooksinamerica.com

Contents

Part 1 My Gluten-Free Knoxville Resources 1
Knoxville's Gluten-Free Food Sources 1
Gluten-Free Good News 1
Gluten-Free Products Available in Knoxville's Mainstream Markets 1
Labeled Gluten-Free 2
National Mainstream Brands 2
Gluten-Free Oats 3
Gluten-Free Beer and Cider 5
Mainstream Gluten-Free Foods 6
Local Food Manufacturers 6
Knoxville Area Markets Carrying Gluten-Free Items 9
Knoxville Area Support Resources 12
Knoxville Area Support Groups 12
Celi-Act Support Group 12
Dietitian Locator 13
Local Dietitians with gluten-free experience 13
Eating Gluten-Free in Restaurants 15
Venturing Forth 15
Restaurant Cards 16
Miss Janet's Gluten-Free Restaurant Guide 16
Restaurant Guide in a Gluten-Free Nutshell 19

Dining Gluten Free in Knoxville	20
Knoxville Area Restaurant Listings	21
Online Sources and Apps for Finding Gluten-Free Restaurants	32
Restaurant Recommendations by the Community	33
Restaurant Tales	34
Going Mainstream	36
Alternative Dining Sources	37
Personal Chefs	37
Getting Personal	37
A Personal Chef in Your Kitchen?	37
The Cost of a Personal Chef	38
Knoxville Area Personal Chefs	39
Caterers and Homemade Takeout	40
Part 2 Coping with Gluten Intolerance	41
Excerpts from Gluten-Free Mainstream America	41
Celebrating the Good Food in Gluten Free	41
Introduction	41
Coping	41
What is Gluten, and How Do You Rid It From Your Life?	42
After Diagnosis	43
Emotions and Reality	44
Ubiquitous Gluten	44
Cross Contamination	44

The Healing Process	45
Good News Foods	45
Helping Others	46
Gluten Free is Good Food	47
Gluten-Free Daily Living Resources	48
Newcomer Pep Talk	48
Toxic Foods	49
Healthful Foods	49
Gluten-Free Oats	49
National Organizations	50
Celiac Disease Foundation	50
Gluten-Intolerance Group of North America	50
National Institutes of Health (NIH)	50
National Digestive Diseases Information Clearinghouse	50
Online Shopping	51
Reference Books & Magazines	51
Gluten-Free Living	51
Living Without	51
Gluten-Free Grocery Shopping Guide	51
The Essential Gluten-Free Grocery Guide	52
The Essential Gluten-Free Restaurant Guide, How and Where to Eat Gluten-Free	52
Celiac Sprue: A Guide Through the Medicine Cabinet, by Marcia Milazzo	52
Celiac Disease, A Hidden Epidemic,	52

Gluten-Free Diet, A Comprehensive Resource Guide 52
Kids with Celiac disease: A Family Guide to Raising Happy, Healthy, Gluten-Free Children, ...52
Gluten-Free 101, Easy, Basic Dishes Without Wheat..52
Online Sources and Apps for Finding Gluten-Free Restaurants 53
How to "Gluten Free" Everything 54
Gluten Free Your Kitchen..54
Gluten Free Your Recipes...55
Author Profile 57
Books by the Author..58

Part 1 My Gluten-Free Knoxville Resources

Knoxville's Gluten-Free Food Sources
Where to Find the Good Stuff

Gluten-Free Good News

Since I travel all over the United States, I have the good fortune to spot trends in marketing. I spend a lot of time in food stores, farmer markets, and whole-foods stores looking for foods that are acceptable to my special diet.

Since 2000, when I was diagnosed, I have seen a positive move in the marketing of gluten-free foods. Every day I am seeing more and more of them on the shelves.

Gluten-Free Products Available in Knoxville's Mainstream Markets

There are excellent guides available to help you find gluten free items in your local mainstream grocery store. For a deliciously enlightening long list of products, you may order a copy of the *The Gluten-Free Grocery Shopping Guide* by Matison & Matison; or *The Essential Gluten-Free Grocery Guide* by Triumph Dining. They are listed earlier in this section. Until you can obtain your purchased guides, the following short list will help you, if you are newly diagnosed. This is just a taste of what is out there. You're going to become an avid label reader.

Remember all fresh produce and fresh unprocessed meats are naturally gluten free. Nothing has been added. Most canned vegetables are gluten free. Read the labels, then call manufacturers. You need to be your own gluten-free advocate. The more manufacturers learn of the increasing demand for gluten-free products, the more we will see them on the shelves. It's a market-driven economy. If it's out there and available to us, we will buy it ... as long as it's tasty as well as gluten free.

Food manufacturers are soon to learn: we are a life-long user. A faithful consumer. Gluten free is here to stay. We're an increasing share of the market, not a diminishing share, as more of us are diagnosed daily. Our gluten-free lifestyle is going mainstream.

A word of warning to you, the consumer: Remember it is your responsibility to contact food and drug manufacturers to check on the product's gluten free status. They may change their ingredients at any time. Before you assume the product you've purchased in the past is gluten free, unless it says gluten free on the label, check to make certain it is.

Labeled Gluten-Free

There are many manufacturers of breads, confections, pastas, crackers, and cereals that are labeled gluten-free. Their names are too numerous to list. Isn't that a happy statement? At the head of my personal-choice list are: The Gluten-Free Pantry, Kinnikinnick Foods, Pamela's, Glutino, and Mary's Gone Crackers. You will soon find your favorites, and you'll find many of them on the shelves of the local stores listed in this section as well as online.

One clear point made to me by many of our local markets, if you can't find a particular favorite on the shelf, just put in a request. Don't be afraid to ask.

*I have no affiliation with any of these product manufacturers, other than the fact that I buy them because I personally like them, and they are gluten free, of course.

National Mainstream Brands
that label gluten free, as of this date of publication. A sampling:

Amy's frozen and jarred products: The products they make that are gluten-free are clearly labeled. They make a line of products that are not gluten free. So read the label carefully.

Arrowhead Mills offers gluten-free in addition to their regular line.

Blue Diamond nut products, such as Nut Thins, are gluten free.

Bob's Red Mill products: They make a gluten-free line in addition to the regular line. So, again, read the labels carefully.

Brown Cow Farm offers gluten-free products: On the lid of the yogurt containers it reads, "Add a brown cow to your gluten-free diet. All of our yogurts (except Fruit & Whole Grains) are now certified gluten-free! But nothing's changed about our delicious taste."

General Mills Rice Chex made its entry into the gluten-free mainstream market a few years ago. The favorable response from the public prompted the company to add a total of seven gluten-free Chex cereals to their line. They are found n the *regular* cereal aisle of your *regular* grocery store Our favorite words "gluten-free" are clearly marked on the boxes. Replacing barley malt with a new formula gave birth to the first General Mills gluten-free product, pushing gluten free into mainstream America. General Mills with its associated companies, now offers more than 300 gluten-free products. I am grateful for the company's commitment to our safety and well being. It makes me smile to think of the bright future of gluten free. The Chex website is www.chex.com/gluten free, which offers gluten-free recipes made with these new products.

General Mills has also introduced a gluten-free **Betty Crocker** line of cookie, cake, and brownie mixes. The line wasn't on our local shelves at printing time, but I have no doubt you'll be seeing it in the baking section of our local stores soon.

Hellmann's Real Mayonnaise. Read the label

Lundberg Family Farms rice products

Mission white corn tortilla products

Nature Made nutritional products

Pillsbury (owned by General Mills) offers a line of gluten-free mixes, including gluten-free pie and pastry crust, chocolate chip cookie dough, and thin crust pizza dough.

Smart Balance Buttery Spread by GFA Brands

Stonyfield Farm lists most of their yogurts, smoothies and soy-yogurts as certified gluten free by the Gluten-Free Certification Organization.

Read the labels.

Gluten-Free Oats

The concern with cross-contamination in oats in the processing and packaging is a valid one. (Cross Contamination, Page 6) Years ago, when I was first diagnosed, oats were definitely off limits because of cross-contamination. It has only been recently that some farms have dedicated special lands to ensure the safety of the oats they produce. Being a lover of fresh, slow-cooked, creamy oatmeal and fresh-baked homemade oatmeal cookies, I was elated to learn I could again eat oats. I know of four manufacturers of gluten-free oats, which are listed below.

Gluten-free oats are grown in gluten-free fields with equipment that is dedicated. The oats are tested every step of the way in processing and packaging.

Be aware that many doctors believe we should "wade into the waters" carefully when introducing oats back into our diets. Some of us may not be able to tolerate oats as well as others. As you would with any new food being introduced into your diet, first ask your doctor or your dietary specialist, then sample a little, see how you tolerate it. Proceed cautiously until you are sure you can handle it.

I followed this procedure of gradually adding oats back into my diet. They're back and they're great.

If you haven't yet found them on the shelves of your favorite gluten-free local supplier, you soon will. Bob's Red Mill has recently added oats to its gluten-free line and is distributed locally. And so is the brand Gluten Free Oats, which is available at Earth Fare. The other brands are available through mail order and online sources.

Bob's Red Mill
bobsredmill.com
1-800-349-2173

Cream Hill Estates
creamhillestates.com
1-866-727-3628

Gluten-Free Oats
glutenfreeoats.com
307-754-2058

Gifts of Nature, Inc.
giftsofnature.net
888-275-0003

Gluten-Free Beer and Cider

Beer has historically been off limits for us. However, in today's market, gluten-free beer has finally arrived. There are a couple of boutique breweries, which I list below. The beers are made with sorghum, rice, or honey, and/or corn. The fact that beer has emerged in the gluten-free food chain is a testament to how manufactures are aware of the growing gluten-free market share. An exclamation point to that statement comes with the announcement that Anheuser-Busch has recently introduced a gluten-free beer called Redbridge. Redbridge is offered at Uno Chicago Grill in Maryville. You can order it with your gluten-free pizza. Gluten-free beer has gone mainstream. Ask your local market to see if they will carry any of these for you:

Redbridge
Anheuser-Busch
Distributed nationwide
www.redbridge.com
1-800-DIAL-BUD

Dragon's Gold
Bards Tale Beer Co.
bardsbeer.com and internetwines.com

Passover Honey
Ramapo Valley Brewery
Kosher
rvbrewery.com

New Grist
Lakefront Brewery
lakefrontbrewery.com
1-800-800-9122

Michelob Ultra Light Cider
offered by Anheuser-Busch
This new entry accompanies the Anheuser-Busch first foray into the gluten-fee market with its Redbridge beer. This new product has ⅓ less calories than other hard ciders with its 120 calories per serving.

Mainstream Gluten-Free Foods
not labeled as gluten-free. A sampling:
Bob Evans Farms products: Read the ingredient list, which is reliable.
Bush's Baked Beans: See the section on Local Tennessee Food Manufacturers for more information.
Chun King Soy Sauce
Dove Chocolates
Frito Lay has good labeling and you can trust the corn chips and potato chips. Call the company for a full gluten-free list.
Kraft Mayonnaise: Read the label for Kraft products. They list all ingredients, so any source of gluten is easily identified.
Land O Lakes Butter
La Choy Soy Sauce
Lactaid Milk
McCormick Spices pure spices, not blends
Newman's Own Salad Dressings
Skippy Peanut Butter

Read the labels.

Local Food Manufacturers
Bush Brothers and Company: Bush's Baked Beans
Here is a local food manufacturer with its thumb on the pulse of consumer needs. I called the Consumer Relations phone number, pressed "3" for ingredient information, and the first message addressed the issue of gluten-free. As of this date only three product lines are *not* gluten-free: Bush's Best Chili Bean

line, Bush's Chili Magic line, and the four varieties of Bush's Homestyle Chili line. Also, all products are casein free, soy free, and made without peanuts or peanut oil. I loved Bush's Baked Beans long before I was diagnosed. What a comfort to learn my favorite treats were safe.
Bush Brothers and Company
PO Box 5233, Dept. C
Knoxville, TN 37950-2330
www.bushbeans.com
Consumer Relations: 865-558-5445

Mayfield Dairy Farms, Athens, TN
While the company doesn't actually test for gluten, it offers a generous list of gluten-free products. What this means is they don't add any gluten to these items. Is there a risk for contamination? I believe, after speaking to the Mayfield consumer affairs representative, and after reading about the company policies, the risk of contamination is minimal, and probably unlikely. That is my opinion only. The logic of their manufacturing methods leads me to that conclusion. It is a personal choice on my part. You need to study the facts and reach your own conclusion.

Every day, at the end of production at Mayfield, the machines are broken down and cleaned thoroughly. Each morning, for example, ice cream production begins with plain flavors, such as vanilla, chocolate, strawberry, cherry. There are no ingredients containing gluten in these plain, uncomplicated flavors. After each flavor ends production, the machine is rinsed, then the next flavor is added. As the day progresses, more complicated mixes go into production. That's when flavors, such as cookie dough, are made. Cookies. Gluten. Obvious. At the end of the day, the machines are sanitized.
The company is straightforward in disclosing its manufacturing process. It clearly states that, while the listed products are gluten free as they are made, according to the data they have on file, products containing gluten are made on the same machine. I believe Mayfield Dairy Farms manufactures products in a conscientious way. You can call or write the company for a list of their gluten-free products and make your own decision from that.
Mayfield Dairy Farms, Inc.
PO Box 310
Athens, TN 37371
423-745-2151
1-800-629-3435

Sweetwater Valley Farm, Philadelphia, TN
Cheese is what this company specializes in. From a mild cheddar to a full-bodied southern cheddar "Hickory Smoke" flavor, you'll find a variety of cheeses to suit any mood. The labels are clearly marked with the ingredients.
Sweetwater Valley Farm
17988 W. Lee Highway
Philadelphia, TN 37846
1-877-862-4322
sweetwatervalley.com

Knoxville Area Markets Carrying Gluten-Free Items

The happy news for those of us living the gluten-free life is that we are rich in local resources for finding gluten-free foods. Gluten free is popping up everywhere, it seems. If you can't find a specific favorite product, ask the market to carry it. Customer input is a valuable tool in shaping what products are available locally. If they know we'll buy it, they will furnish it.

    The food industry is aware that this market is an expanding market, not a diminishing one, because more of us are being diagnosed with celiac disease every day. Gluten-free living is a life-long commitment. As food producers recognize our market share, we will be seeing even a greater variety of delicious gluten-free products on our local grocery store shelves. The variety of gluten-free products are already increasing at a dizzying rate over what was available only a few years ago. It is a positive, welcome trend.

    The following stores carry a few of the same products, and some carry more varieties than others. I find all these stores have something of value and interest. I applaud their efforts to address the needs of our gluten-free community. I expect this reference section to grow with each edition of the book. If you know of other local gluten-free food sources, please share that information with me. I'll pass it along.

Apple Tree
729 Louisville Rd.
Alcoa (next door to Panera Bread)
865-977-110

Benefit Your Life
Natural Lifestyle Market
620 N. Campbell Station Road, Suite 24
Knoxville, TN 37934
865-288-3193
benefityourlifestore.com

Butler & Bailey Market
7513 South Northshore Drive
Knoxville, TN 37919
(865) 694-9045

My Gluten-Free Knoxville

Earth Fare *Also referenced in the Restaurant Listings*
You will find a literal gluten-free paradise offering many gluten-free selections, which are marked in each section of the store. Look for the signs "gluten-free." And look for small marks of "G.F." on tags in various sections. Some gluten-free products are now available in the deli/cafe section, including fresh gluten-free cake. The ingredients are listed on all the store-made deli items. If you wish to order gluten-free pasta salad or macaroni and cheese, call ahead of time to order.

Earth Fare *Also referenced in the Restaurant Listings*
10903 Parkside Drive (Turkey Creek)
Knoxville, TN
865-777-3837
            and
140 North Forest Park
Knoxville, TN 37919
865-558-1432
earthfare.com

The Epicurean
43 E. Tennessee Avenue
Oak Ridge, TN
865-483-1541

Food City - all locations
foodcity.com

Go Nutrition
10961 Kingston Pike
Knoxville, TN
865-675-8886

Ingles Market
11847 Kingston Pike
Knoxville, TN 37934
865-966-4360

Kroger Markets - all locations
Kroger Markets carries a variety of quality gluten-free products. Many are located in the natural foods section.
kroger.com

Three Rivers Market
(formerly called the Food Co-op)
They offer a small, basic selection.
937 Broadway
Knoxville, TN
525-2069

Publix Market - all locations
publix.com

Trader Joe's
8001 Kingston Pike
Knoxville, TN 37919
865-670-4088
traderjoes.com

WalMart - all locations
Each WalMart is a little different. Check out various stores in your area to find the one that suits your gluten-free needs the best. Some carry more gluten-free items than others.
walmart.com

Whole Foods Market
(slated for a store opening in West Knoxville soon)
wholefoodsmarket.com

Knoxville Area Support Resources

Knoxville Area Support Groups

If there isn't a support group in your area, start one. It's easy. Contact the Gluten Intolerance Group (listed in the Daily Living Resource section) for more information on how to get started. If there are only two of you with celiac disease in your area, at least you are two neighbors with much in common. It doesn't have to be a formal organization. Get together now and then to compare notes, have tea, share recipes, talk shop about doctors, health issues, latest news in research, where to find good fresh gluten-free ingredients, and share coping techniques. Keep in touch. With one in 133 Americans having celiac disease, your group is sure to grow.

As of this date, I am aware of only one gluten-free group in the Knoxville area. If you know of others, or if you start your own, please notify me and I will pass along the information in my next edition of this guide.

Celi-Act Support Group

The Children's Hospital Pediatric Gastroenterology has a website www.giforkids.com. You'll find helpful information, including the support group called CELI-ACT.

The support group has its own website: www.celi-act.com. There you'll learn of their upcoming events and support group meetings. Adults, as well as children, are welcome in this group. It is open to anyone and everyone associated with celiac disease.

Celiac-disease and the gluten-free lifestyle is often a family affair. Once one member of the family has celiac disease, there are often others in the family with it, as well. Even grandparents are coming to meetings to learn about what they can have on hand in their homes to safely offer their recently diagnosed grandchildren.

The group, that is expanding, meets every other month on the third Monday at 6 p.m. They usually meet in the Menschendorf Conference Room, Koppel Plaza, at the East Tennessee Children's Hospital.

This is an active, highly motivated group. Every year, the group organizes a phenomenal event, the Celi-Act Gluten-Free Vendor Fair. My hats off to this group. Great job creating awareness for our gluten-intolerant community!

Dietitian Locator
Local Dietitians with gluten-free experience

Your dietitian can answer your questions with good scientific fact, advice, personalized menus, and basically help you along the path to good nutritional health. Since a strict adherence to a gluten-free diet is the only treatment for celiac disease, it's important to maintain a balanced diet geared to our specific needs. A registered dietitian is on the front-line of our battle to regain and maintain our health.

One way to locate a dietitian is through the American Dietetic Association. The American Dietetic Association has gluten-free guidelines, which are well distributed throughout the association. Look online at www.eatright.org:

You can also find a nutrition professional in the Knoxville area phone book under Dietitians. The professionals listed below are knowledgeable about gluten-free diets. When you call to make an appointment with a dietary specialist, ask about experience with celiac disease. Ask about local support groups. It has been my observation that dietitians always seem to have a good "thumb-on-the-pulse" of the needs of their communities.

Sandy Altizer, RD, LDN
Specializing in Celiac Disease and the Gluten Free Diet
GI for Kids, PLLC
Children's Hospital Medical Office Building
2100 Clinch Avenue
MOB, Suite 510
Knoxville, TN 37916
865.546.3998, ext. 290
865.329.3204 (fax)
www.giforkids.com

Becky Burnett, RN, LDN
Children's Hospital
2018 Clinch Ave.
Knoxville, TN 37916
865-541-8512

Heather Kaufman, RD, LDN
University Internal Medicine and Integrative Health
1932 Alcoa Hwy
Knoxville, TN 37920
865-971-3539

Callie Jubran, RD, LDN
GI for Kids, PLLC
2100 Clinch Avenue Suite 510
Knoxville, TN 37916
(865) 546-3998

Jennifer Masters, MS, RD, LDN, Certified LEAP Therapist
Pediatric Dietary Specialists
Pediatric Gastroenterology & Nutritional Support, P.C.
2100 W. Clinch Ave., Suite 230
Knoxville, TN 37922
865-522-4116

Janet Seiber, RD, LDN, CDE
The University of Tennessee Medical Center
Wellness Nutrition
Healthcare Coordination: 865-305-6970

Ashley Rogers Treadway, MS, RD, LDN
GI for Kids, PLLC
2100 Clinch Avenue Suite 510
Knoxville, TN 37916
(865) 546-3998

Eating Gluten-Free in Restaurants
Venturing Forth

After I was first diagnosed, I would not eat in a restaurant for more than a year. I felt that toxins lurked outside the safety of my gluten-free zone, and I was reluctant to venture forth. But my story has a happy ending. Slowly and cautiously I have found many fine chefs around the country who care about my food restrictions and want to provide me with a good dining experience. Caring is the first step, education is the second. I have my favorite restaurants now where I can enjoy an excellent meal as normally as I used to before I became ill. I continue to expand my envelope of safety to include other good restaurants, which I know are many. And I am doing it one chef at a time.

Most of the time I have the luxury of knowing ahead of time where we're dining, and I speak to the chef a couple of days before I arrive. I try to call at a time of day that won't conflict with lunch or dinner preparations. If the chef is new to gluten-free cooking, I explain my dietary restrictions and we go over the menu. We talk about ingredients and about safe food preparation, cross contamination, and the necessity of alerting the kitchen staff to be aware. Even a small amount of gluten is toxic to those of us with celiac disease. The chef and I usually decide ahead of time what I will be served so on the night of our reservations there is no fuss. When I arrive, they are ready for me, and I can enjoy my evening without worry.

There are times when it is impossible to know in advance of our dinner arrangements. If it is an upscale restaurant, I am usually able to find something on the menu that can be adapted to my needs, even if it's a simple non-marinated grilled steak, baked potato, and garden salad ("no croutons, please") with oil and vinegar. It's good, it's fresh, and it's safe.

To some social events in restaurants I will take my own food, or not eat at all, rather than risk being poisoned. I won't eat at large banquets, or at fast-food places, for example — any place where the frazzled wait staff is much too busy to worry about the lady at table eight who is on a diet with a weird name. "Would you like a roll with that, ma'am?"

When I am building a trusted relationship with a new chef, I share my personal experiences of dining out. Most of them are good experiences, however, some of them have been horror stories where gluten shows up on my plate in spite of everyone's best intentions. It helps a chef to know that a large majority of us who are newly diagnosed are afraid of being poisoned in restaurants because of lack of awareness and understanding of proper food preparation and the seriousness of our requirements. If we can be assured that everything possible is being done to make our food source safe, we will begin to eat out again. That is why a Gluten-Free Awareness Campaign is so important. Restaurant owners need to know they have a large untapped resource of potential and loyal customers.

Restaurant Cards

A Restaurant Card contains information about your gluten-free requirements. It is an efficient way to inform a chef and the kitchen staff of your specific needs, and at the same time, it lets them know that this is a serious issue. You will find restaurant cards on most websites and in all books focusing on the subject of dining gluten free. They are convenient guides for anyone preparing you a gluten-free meal. You can laminate a card and carry it with you wherever you go. Carry a spare in case your server forgets to give it back to you.

    I have included my Gluten-free Awareness Campaign brochure in this guide. It's my version of a Restaurant Card. It not only explains what is toxic and what is gluten free, but it mentions the importance of dedicated cooking utensils, cross contamination factors, and even lists websites where the chef can obtain more information. Make photocopies of it and take it along with you every single time you eat out. Give it to the chef or your server. Tell them they can keep it, and then leave it behind. Spread the word. I've been to several restaurants where I've announced that I'm on a medically restricted diet and my meal must be gluten free. A server will say, "Well, we have a brochure on that posted in the kitchen." It turns out to be one I left there several months ago. That is proof that the good folks in the restaurant business are caring and concerned for our well being. I love it when that happens.

    I always leave my gluten-free awareness campaign brochure with the staff. I've had chefs come out from their kitchens to tell me how much they appreciated the brochure. One of them said it was good to have something with references so he could learn more about the diet. Another one said the information was valuable because, "it tells me not only what you can't eat, but it tells me what you can eat."

Miss Janet's Gluten-Free Restaurant Guide

The following brochure is a crash course on how to cook gluten free for restaurant owners, chefs and staff. The brochure also directs them to trusted websites so they may continue their education. Photo copy the brochure, front and back, on the following two pages, yielding two guides per page. Take copies with you wherever you go. This is good news that we like to share.

My Gluten-Free Knoxville

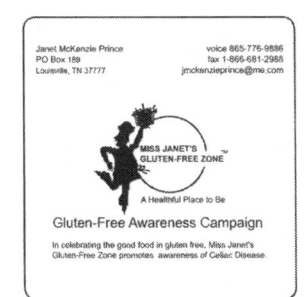

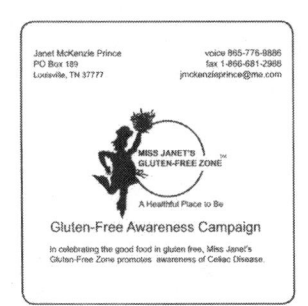

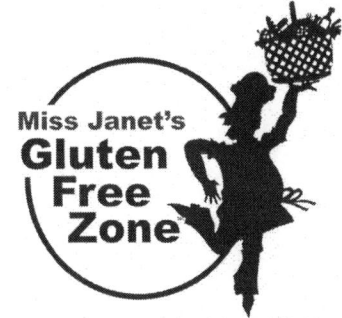

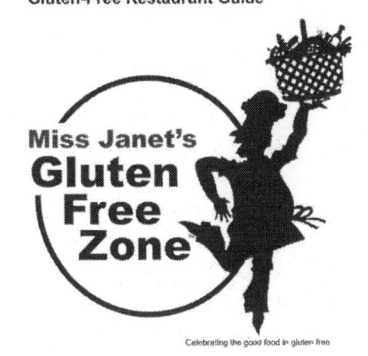

My Gluten-Free Knoxville

Gluten Free
A Medically Required Diet
for Celiac Disease

A Gluten-Free diet is a medically required diet for people with Celiac Disease. According to recent studies, one in 133 Americans are affected.

What is Celiac Disease?
It is an inherited autoimmune disease. The immune system reacts to the ingestion gluten found in wheat, rye, and barley and their derivatives. (Oats are suspect because of cross contamination in growing and processing.) The toxin sets off an autoimmune reaction that damages the lining of the small intestine, blocking the absorption of nutrients. It is a life-long, non-curable sensitivity. It can be controlled through strict adherence to a gluten-free diet.

Gluten-Free Forever
The gluten-free diet is a diet for life. Those of us with Celiac Disease do not have a choice to eat or not to eat foods containing gluten. We must not ingest any form of wheat, rye, or barley to avoid serious intestinal damage.

The Good-News Diet
Because of the freshness of our foods and the avoidance of processed foods, our diet is a healthful diet for everyone.

One in 133 Americans have Celiac Disease. It is twice as common as Crohn's disease, ulcerative colitis, and cystic fibrosis combined. Comparatively, one million Americans have Parkinson's disease. More than 3 million Americans are affected by Celiac Disease. In addition, when we include those with non-celiac gluten intolerance, our ranks expand to 15 million.

Toxic Foods
Gluten is a toxic protein found in wheat, rye, and barley. Avoid all derivatives of these grains, including spelt, kamut, triticale. Toxins are in wheat pasta (remember semolina is from wheat), graham, bulgur, wheat germ, and sauces, gravies, and marinades using flour thickeners. Avoid breaded coatings, croutons, malt, hydrolyzed wheat protein, or modified wheat starch. Beware of French fried potatoes prepared in the same oil as breaded fried chicken and onion rings, for example. Gluten may also present in oats due to cross contamination if not grown and processed in a dedicated gluten-free environment. Even a small amount of gluten will damage the intestines.

Healthful Foods
We can eat all fresh, non-processed vegetables. Safe foods include potatoes, roots and tubers, rice (white, brown, wild), corn, sorghum, tapioca, buckwheat (good grain, bad name), amaranth, quinoa, millet and teff. All fresh, non-processed meats, poultry, fish, beans, legumes, and nuts are healthful. Eggs are safe as well as milk, many cheeses, some yogurts, and pure butter. Oils and vinegars are safe. Avoid processed foods. Fresh is Best.

In Food Preparation
Protection against cross-contamination is a key ingredient in the gluten-free diet. All cooking surfaces and utensils must be clean and separate.

Sources for Further Information
The Gluten Intolerance Group of North America www.gluten.net
Gluten Free Certification Organization www.gfco.org
Gluten Free Restaurant Awareness Program www.glutenfreerestaurants.org
The Celiac Disease Foundation www.celiac.org

Gluten Free
A Medically Required Diet
for Celiac Disease

A Gluten-Free diet is a medically required diet for people with Celiac Disease. According to recent studies, one in 133 Americans are affected.

What is Celiac Disease?
It is an inherited autoimmune disease. The immune system reacts to the ingestion gluten found in wheat, rye, and barley and their derivatives. (Oats are suspect because of cross contamination in growing and processing.) The toxin sets off an autoimmune reaction that damages the lining of the small intestine, blocking the absorption of nutrients. It is a life-long, non-curable sensitivity. It can be controlled through strict adherence to a gluten-free diet.

Gluten-Free Forever
The gluten-free diet is a diet for life. Those of us with Celiac Disease do not have a choice to eat or not to eat foods containing gluten. We must not ingest any form of wheat, rye, or barley to avoid serious intestinal damage.

The Good-News Diet
Because of the freshness of our foods and the avoidance of processed foods, our diet is a healthful diet for everyone.

One in 133 Americans have Celiac Disease. It is twice as common as Crohn's disease, ulcerative colitis, and cystic fibrosis combined. Comparatively, one million Americans have Parkinson's disease. More than 3 million Americans are affected by Celiac Disease. In addition, when we include those with non-celiac gluten intolerance, our ranks expand to 15 million.

Toxic Foods
Gluten is a toxic protein found in wheat, rye, and barley. Avoid all derivatives of these grains, including spelt, kamut, triticale. Toxins are in wheat pasta (remember semolina is from wheat), graham, bulgur, wheat germ, and sauces, gravies, and marinades using flour thickeners. Avoid breaded coatings, croutons, malt, hydrolyzed wheat protein, or modified wheat starch. Beware of French fried potatoes prepared in the same oil as breaded fried chicken and onion rings, for example. Gluten may also present in oats due to cross contamination if not grown and processed in a dedicated gluten-free environment. Even a small amount of gluten will damage the intestines.

Healthful Foods
We can eat all fresh, non-processed vegetables. Safe foods include potatoes, roots and tubers, rice (white, brown, wild), corn, sorghum, tapioca, buckwheat (good grain, bad name), amaranth, quinoa, millet and teff. All fresh, non-processed meats, poultry, fish, beans, legumes, and nuts are healthful. Eggs are safe as well as milk, many cheeses, some yogurts, and pure butter. Oils and vinegars are safe. Avoid processed foods. Fresh is Best.

In Food Preparation
Protection against cross-contamination is a key ingredient in the gluten-free diet. All cooking surfaces and utensils must be clean and separate.

Sources for Further Information
The Gluten Intolerance Group of North America www.gluten.net
Gluten Free Certification Organization www.gfco.org
Gluten Free Restaurant Awareness Program www.glutenfreerestaurants.org
The Celiac Disease Foundation www.celiac.org

Restaurant Guide in a Gluten-Free Nutshell

Call in advance. Don't call during peak hours. Talk to the chef, the food manager, or the owner. Ask questions and be prepared to answer all of theirs. Discuss what is on your Restaurant Card. Give them a mini-course on gluten-free requirements and issues of cross contamination. Plain, fresh food is a place to start. Only when you are sure they understand the issue of gluten-free, then let them add their own natural, fresh ingredients for sauces and garnishes.

If you have favorite restaurants that cater to your gluten-free needs, please write to me with your comments. My address is at the end of this guide.

Dining Gluten Free in Knoxville

Who is cooking gluten free in Knoxville? My list is growing daily, I'm happy to say. I'm on a search-and-enjoy gluten-free mission.

It gives me great pleasure to share my experiences about dining gluten-free in Knoxville. Since I travel frequently, I've had the good fortune to be pampered by several top-notch chefs around the country. Each has risen to the occasion to ensure the food prepared for me is safe as well as delicious. I'm finding more and more chefs who are familiar with the gluten-free requirements of celiac disease. Those who are not familiar with the dietary restrictions of celiac disease are eager to learn. The chefs I have met take the gluten-free challenge seriously, and they have never let me down.

Locally, we have several fine restaurants that are aware of the needs of their gluten-free clients. Our gluten-free community is growing, and so is the concern and caring from the restaurants that serve those of us with celiac disease.

One caveat that I will share with you, which is a truism no matter what the source of recommendation: **On any given day, something that was recommended may not be up to par the next day. There are no guarantees.** I can recommend these establishments for their gluten-free aptitude and my successes with them, but I cannot guarantee that they will always be gluten free, because I cannot make that claim for them. You must ask your own questions and make your decision based on your findings.

Be Aware
Assume nothing
Verify everything

Chefs are food enthusiasts. They love to share their passion with others. They rise to the challenge of providing safe and delicious meals for all who enter their establishments. Those of us with dietary restrictions owe it to these dedicated chefs to communicate our needs so they can continue their good works. We reap the benefits, and everyone goes home a winner.

Knoxville Area Restaurant Listings

Bear with me as I walk you though this disclaimer. Restaurants come and go. New restaurants open up. Some close their doors after a few months or a few years. Restaurant managers change. Chefs move to other restaurants, or move out of state. This list is current as of this writing. It may change tomorrow. Certainly, as time goes on, more restaurants will offer gluten free. Therefore, this list will always be incomplete.

Knowing that things will change, before you go, please check with the management to see if they are still there and are still able to accommodate a gluten-free diet.

Most restaurants do not have gluten-free kitchens, but are well informed and make every attempt to accommodate our special needs. I support their efforts to keep us safe. You still must do your own investigation if you wish to eat there, ask questions, and make your own decision. The more we promote gluten-free awareness, the safer our food supply will be.

Abuelos - gluten-free menu
Turkey Creek Colonial Pinnacle
11299 Parkside Dr.
Knoxville, TN 37934
865-966-0075
abuelos.com

Aubrey's - gluten-free menu
Aubrey's has several locations throughout the area. Please go to the website for a complete list.
102 South Campbell Station Road
Knoxville, TN
865-671-2233
    and
Located behind the Landmark Towers on the corner of Northshore Drive and Papermill Road
6005 Brookvale Lane
Knoxville, TN
865-588-1111
    and

Aubrey's (continued)
481 S. Illinois Avenue
Oak Ridge, TN
865-685-0821
aubreysrestaurants.com

Bonefish Grill – gluten-free menu
11395 Parkside Dr. (at Turkey Creek)
Knoxville, TN
865-966-9777
    and
6610 Kingston Pike (Bearden)
Knoxville, TN
865-558-5743
bonefishgrill.com

Café 4 at Market Square - gluten-free menu
4 Market Square SW
Knoxville, TN
cafe4ms.com
865-544-4144

Calhoun's on the River
400 Neyland Dr.
Knoxville, TN
865-288-1600

Cherokee Country Club (Members-Only Private Club)
5138 Lyons View Pike
Knoxville, TN
865-584-4637

Chili's – gluten-free menu
chilis.com for a gluten-free menu download "allergen information" with wise advice: "prior to placing your order, please always alert the manager to your food allergy or special dietary needs."
Chili's has numerous locations in the Knoxville area including Alcoa, North Knoxville, Lenoir City.

Chop House
9700 Kingston Pike
Knoxville, TN
865-531-2467
Connor Concepts Inc, with several restaurants in the company's chain, has been exposed to my gluten-free awareness campaign. I've had fine meals at The Chop House on Kingston Pike and at Connors Steak House and Seafood at Turkey Creek.

Connor's Steak & Seafood
10915 Turkey Dr. (Turkey Creek)
Knoxville, TN
865-966-0933

Cru Bistro and Wine Bar- gluten-free menu
11383 Parkside Dr. (Turkey Creek)
Knoxville, TN 37934
865-671-6612
          and
141 South Gay St. (Downtown)
Knoxville, TN 37901
865-544-1491
crubistroandwinebar.com

Earth Fare Deli & Café *Also referenced in the Market Listings*
10903 Parkside Drive (Turkey Creek)
Knoxville, TN
865-777-3837
        and
140 North Forest Park
Knoxville, TN 37919
865-558-1432
earthfare.com
This is a worthwhile destination even if you don't have any grocery shopping to do. The fresh rotisserie chicken is gluten free, as well as many other deli items. All the ingredients are listed for everything they make. Take it out or eat it there.

Echo Bistro and Wine Bar
5803 Kingston Pike (Homberg)
Knoxville, TN
865-602-2090
When you make your reservations, note you are gluten free. Both owners,

Five Guys
There are several locations in our area. Go online for the complete list.
Five Guys Burgers & Fries
208 Hamilton Crossing Dr.
Alcoa, TN 37701
865-982-1200
        and
Five Guys Famous Burgers
10922 Parkside Dr.
Knoxville, TN
865-675-4897
fiveguys.com
Obviously, order the burger without the bun. They toast the bread on a separate grill from the one used for the meat patties. But I would ask the manager to be certain. They claim the fries are safe because the use plain potatoes cooked in peanut oil and nothing else is fried in that oil.

Fleming's Steakhouse
11287 Parkside Dr. (Turkey Creek)
Knoxville, TN
865-675-9463

Foothills Milling Company
315 S. Washington St.
Maryville, TN
865-977-8434
foothillsmillingcompany.com
The **Foothills Milling Company** in Maryville speaks gluten free. It is another comfort zone for me. When you call ahead to make a reservation, tell them you require gluten free and they will go out of their way to help you. Owners Tommy Vaughan, manager, and Bart Vaughan, executive chef, run a fine establishment.

Fox Den Country Club (Members-Only Private Club)
12284 North Fox Den Dr.
Knoxville, TN
865-675-5260
If you are a member, or a guest of a member, you should still call ahead and alert the staff to your specific needs.

Jason's Deli - gluten-free menu
A national chain with two Knoxville locations.
Go to the website and order the iPhone or iPad app for ordering before you arrive.
133 N Peters Rd
Knoxville, TN 37923
    and
2120 Cumberland Ave
Knoxville, TN 37916
jasonsdeli.com

My Gluten-Free Knoxville

Lakeside Tavern
off Northshore Drive
10911 Concord Park Dr.
Knoxville, TN
865-671-2980

Longhorn Steakhouse (opened in Fall of 2012)
11644 Parkside Dr. (Turkey Creek)
Knoxville, TN 37934
865-966-6954
longhornsteakhouse.com
They have what they call a "gluten-sensitive menu" that you can find online. I've eaten at several Longhorn locations in other cities and have had great success due to their well informed staff.

Mellow Mushroom
2109 Cumberland Ave.,
Knoxville, TN 37916
865-687-4766
      and
635 N. Campbell Station Rd.
Farragut, TN 37934
mellowmushroom.com

Mimi's Café
110945 Parkside Dr. (Turkey Creek)
Knoxville, TN
865-675-1362

Moe's Southwest Grill
1800 Cumberland Avenue
Knoxville, TN 37916
865-637-2700
      and
9450 South Northshore Dr.
Knoxville, TN 37922
865-470-2844
      and
11322 Parkside Dr.
Knoxville, TN 37934
865-675-6637
download their allergen chart at
moes.com

Mulligans Restaurant at Gettysvue Center
8923 Linksvue Dr
Knoxville, TN 37922
865-862-8923
eatatmulligans.com
Call ahead if you can. Talk to owner Don Anderson. Don and his wife Patti will take you through their menu. They will go out of their way to accommodate gluten free requests.

Northshore Brasserie
9430 S. Northshore Dr.
Knoxville, TN
(near Pellissippi at Lakeside Village)
865-539-5188
www.northshorebrasserie.com

The Northshore Brasserie, with its French & Belgian cuisine, is a comfort zone for me. There are items on the menu with naturally gluten free ingredients in the entrees and salads. It is always best to call ahead with your gluten-free reservation, however, I often just pop in with the assurance that I'll find a comforting meal that I can order right off the menu. Owned by two brothers and their sister, Brian, Russell, and Stephanie Balest, the restaurant offers a casual setting with delicious food under the careful guidance of Executive Chef Jesse Newmister.

O'Charley's (a chain with several locations around town, including Alcoa and Turkey Creek)
www.ocharleys.com
They offer an ingredient listing that tells you what ingredients are in each dish. Ask your questions carefully to be sure the staff truly understands your specific requirements.

Orangery
5412 Kingston Pike
Knoxville, TN
865-588-2964
When you make your reservation, state you are gluten free and make it well known when you arrive at your table.

Oriental Cuisine
622 Condry Lane
Maryville, TN 37803
865-984-0810
Before you go for the first time, call the manager, Mi Mi, to satisfy yourself that they understand the concept of cross-contamination and gluten-free food preparation. They do not have a specific gluten-free menu, but they can adapt many dishes to your needs. They do have a gluten-free soy sauce available. When I visited the restaurant, Mi Mi and her staff gave me the confidence that they could prepare a safe meal for me, and they did. They have several gluten-free families who visit on a regular basis. They serve American, Chinese, Tai, and Vietnamese foods.

Outback Steak House – national gluten-free menu
Several locations around town
outbacksteakhouse.com

Petro's Chili & Chips
www.petros.com
Numerous locations around Knoxville and Oak Ridge.
I called the corporate headquarters about their ingredients. The Petro is gluten free. Most everything else should be gluten free. But the wrap (if made with flour) is not gluten free. Nor is the pasta dish. Ask questions before your order.
1033 North Cedar Bluff Rd.
Knoxville, TN 37923
865-690-2920

Pei Wei Asian Diner - national gluten-free menu
11301 Parkside Dr., Suite 1200 (Turkey Creek)
Knoxville, TN 37901
865-966-1610
peiweiasiandiner.com

My Gluten-Free Knoxville

P.F. Chang's - national gluten-free menu
6741 Kingston Pike
Knoxville, TN
865-212-5514
pfchangs.com

Rouxbarb's
130 S. Northshore
Knoxville, TN
865-212-0024
Chef Bruce Bogartz understands gluten free in his restaurant and in his catering business.

Ruth's Chris Steakhouse – gluten-free menu
950 Volunteer Landing Ln
Knoxville, TN 37915-2594
(865) 546-4696
Your gluten-free request will be met by a savvy, competent staff that has been trained in all aspects of cooking gluten free.

Season's Grill - gluten-free menu
12740 Kingston Pike, Suite 106
Renaissance Center (Farragut)
Knoxville, TN
865-671-3679
              and
5018 Kingston Pike (Bearden)
Knoxville, TN
865-766-5331

Season's Café owner and Executive Chef Deron Little embraces the Gluten-Free Zone concept. For his ever-increasing patrons living the gluten-free life, he offers a gluten-free menu and keeps gluten-free breads in the freezer in case we're simply in the mood for something as uncomplicated as a sandwich.

Something Savory Bakery & Café
541 High Street
Maryville, TN 37804
865-984-0550

The Tomato Head
12 Market Square
Knoxville, TN 37902
865-637-4067
            and
7240 Kingston Pike, Suite 172
Knoxville, TN 37919
865-584-1078
thetomatohead.com
Both locations offer catering, a café, and take out. You will find a refreshingly fresh healthful menu, and gluten-free is spoken there. No gluten-free menu, but they offer many items that you can substitute with corn tortillas.

National Chains
National chains are increasingly addressing the needs of the gluten-free community. Our local **P.F.Chang's** is extremely knowledgeable in gluten-free cooking. They even provide a special gluten-free menu, as does **Bonefish Grill, Chili's,** and **Outback Steakhouse**. **Mimi's Café**, and **Fleming's Steakhouse** also offer specific gluten-free information.
    Many fast-food chains offer gluten-free items. Always ask questions to satisfy yourself if the food is safe from cross contamination. Ask what is cooked in separate fryers. Check out their sanitation policies, such as changing gloves before preparing your gluten-free item. This is just a sampling of the chains that say they offer gluten-free: **Wendy's, Sonic, Burger King, Chick-fil-A, Chipotle Mexican Grill, In-N-Out Burger,** and **Dairy Queen**.

Online Sources and Apps for Finding Gluten-Free Restaurants

Mobile apps and online sources are cropping up daily. This is just a sampling. Some are free apps, and some cost a few dollars. Go to the websites to download the apps.

Gluten-Free Restaurant Awareness Program: glutenfreerestaurants.org

Gluten-Free Dining Guide: celiacrestaurantguide.com

DineGF: Gluten-free chain restaurant menus and locations: glutenfreetravelsite.com

Locate all things gluten free near you: glutenfreeregistry.com

Yelp. Type in gluten-free restaurants in the search window: yelp.com

Locate allergy friendly restaurants near you: allergyeats.com

Locate chain restaurants, local restaurants, recipes and products: findmeglutenfree.com

Chain restaurants with gluten-free and allergen lists, custom to your needs:
glutenfreepassport.com: iCanEat OnTheGo Gluten Free & Allergen Free. Another app gives you information on ethnic restaurant ingredients: iEatOut Gluten & Allergen Free

celiac-disease.com. Click on the Restaurant tab. Choose your state. It also lists local grocery stores.

Restaurant Recommendations by the Community

This is a new section listing restaurant recommendations from our local gluten-free community. I encourage community involvement with this guide. Please make this guide your own. Give me your personal recommendations. Get involved. My goal is to have everyone say with pride, "This is my gluten-free Knoxville."

I have no personal experience with these establishments at this time. Now they are on my list of new places to try. Thanks to those who contributed.

The Soup Kitchen
Cedar Springs Center
9222 Kingston Pike
Knoxville, TN
865-705-8580

T.C.'S Grille
732 Calderwood Hwy.
Maryville, TN 37801
Owner Shirley Clark

Tellico Harbor Restaurant
1000 Marina Harbour Dr.
Maryville, TN 37801
865-856-9059

Restaurant Tales

Don't be Afraid. Just be Careful.
You'll soon have tales of your own to relate. Restaurant dining should be pleasant and risk free. On rare occasions dining has been a little stressful for me. Now that I'm a seasoned gluten-free adventurer, I can put these stories in perspective. When gluten appears on your plate, expect all sorts of reactions. Here are a few snippets from my experiences.

In Maryland:
A phone conversation: "May I talk to the chef?" I asked. "I'm on a medically restricted diet that must be gluten free, and I'd like to talk to him about it."

"Well, he's pretty tied up at the moment. Let me just tell him about it, okay?'
Moments later the fellow returns to the phone. "Okay! We gottcha covered. The chef knows all about it! He's dealt with this before."

"Well, that's happy news. What does he know?"

"No eggs, no milk, no chicken."

In Arizona:
After detailed explanations to the server, and after giving her my restaurant card to take to the chef, she assured me she understood completely.

"My cousin has that problem. I know all about it."

"Nothing touching my food. No wheat. No bread. No croutons. Really. Cross contamination is a big problem."

"Yep!" She soon returned to the table with a salad capped proudly with a soft, fresh dinner roll. When I pointed out the obvious fact that the roll sitting on my salad was made with toxic wheat flour, she tartly said, "Oh, no problem!" She then reached across the table to my plate, snatched the roll from atop the salad, and plunked it down on the table. "There! All better!"

In California:
The server was completely attentive. He took my restaurant card to the chef, and everyone seemed to be on top of my gluten-free theme at this upscale restaurant in Pasadena. "I'll prepare your salad myself," he said. When he delivered our salads, mine was laden with croutons. My husband noticed it before I did.

"Her salad is crawling with croutons!"

The server froze. His face turned red. "I am SO sorry!" His embarrassment made me feel so sorry for him. "I lost my concentration! I am soooo sorry! I knew better than that." I told him to just skip the salad and I'd just wait for my dinner. He'd have none of that. "No, no! I'll fix it for you myself. I won't let you down again."

The second salad was gluten free. And my magnificent gluten-free meal of steak and steamed vegetables that evening was gratis, compliments of the management.

In Tennessee:
I was dining at a restaurant that offers a gluten-free menu. I placed my order, and my brother ordered gluten-free as well. He does not have celiac disease, but wanted to see what the experience was like in a restaurant for me. When his meal was served, I asked in astonishment, "What type of noodles are these? They don't look like the rice noodles that I have had in the past." Sure enough, they were egg noodles made with wheat flour. The lesson there is to question everything, even where they have a gluten-free menu. Ordering gluten free doesn't guarantee you'll get gluten free. When in doubt, don't eat it. My brother was impressed with the uncertainties I face every time I eat out. And when his meal was served the second time, it was gluten-free and delicious.

In Arizona:
While visiting Tucson, we hosted a party at a restaurant because the chef and his staff were in tune with my special diet. I had eaten there several times that week. In fact, I hosted a luncheon for my friends a few days before.

The waiter was new...all smiles and eager to do a good job for this large group. He was aware that we were having dinner there because of me. My choice. We could go anywhere in this food-culturally-rich city, and we chose this one because I trusted the staff. They understood the gluten-free regime.

As we were being served our salads, conversation at our table stopped abruptly when my friend across the table shouted, "Don't touch that salad!" My husband had reacted at the same time, also warning me, and pulled my salad away from me. "Croutons! Croutons? Croutons are toxic to her!" This is yet another example of a server, who said he understood, but completely didn't. It's also an example of never being able to let down your guard, even when you think you're in a safe environment. I often refer to this incident as my "It-Takes-a-Village" experience. I have a wide safety net of friends and family. I am comforted by their caring, protective, all-embracing concern for my well-being.

Going Mainstream

I listed these few stories just to give you a taste of the real world. Don't be afraid, just be careful. The joys of gluten-free restaurant dining far out weigh the few glitches you may find along the way. We must prevail. We must keep venturing into mainstream restaurants with our positive expectations. We must educate chefs, we must keep spreading the word from food managers to food servers. As we bring our diet out into the open on a regular basis, it will filter into the mainstream.

    It won't be long before we can walk into any restaurant and order a gluten-free meal without it being an issue. I'm finding that in local restaurants I frequent around Knoxville as well as restaurants around the United States, as I travel. On one of my trips to California I located a delightful small restaurant in Santa Rosa. I called to make a reservation and to talk to the chef. I was prepared to go into great detail about my medically restricted diet, when I learned she knew about the diet and had prepared gluten-free meals in the past. The small dinner party I arranged was a success and I had a fabulous gluten-free meal that I enjoyed as much as my guests enjoyed their meals. That's the way it should be. A normal dining experience. Mainstream.

    So, my friends, get out there and order gluten free!

Alternative Dining Sources
Personal Chefs

Getting Personal

Interviewing personal chefs has been another fun adventure for me. In Maryland, where we lived before coming to East Tennessee, I had an excellent personal chef who was fluent in gluten-free.

We first met Mitch Greene through friends in Columbia, South Carolina. It was a special occasion at their home, and Chef Mitch was in the kitchen whipping up wonderful things. His mission for that evening was to prepare a totally gluten-free meal for eight diners. The hosts were kind enough to ensure nothing in their home that night was off limits to me. They sterilized counters and cooking surfaces and pots and pans. I was the only one with celiac disease. But everyone would be eating gluten free. It was an extreme honor for me to be treated with such loving care.

When I first walked in the door, aromas of focaccia tickled my nose. I hadn't tasted focaccia for years. It's not that easy to make gluten free focaccia. This was years before the mixes came out, and Mitch wouldn't use a mix anyway. This was made-from-scratch fresh gluten-free bread. He served it as an appetizer and received nothing but praise from the other guests, who had never tasted gluten-free anything before.

Of course, my rating of Mitch's efforts for the evening was over the top! Mitch cooked for me again a few months later at a large gathering at a prestigious private club in Columbia, SC. This time he wasn't the head chef, because the club had its own chef. Mitch came in and personally delivered a very special gluten-free dinner for me. "Madam, Chef Mitch has arrived with your gluten-free meal." Heads turned. "Excuse me, how can we get what she's eating?" Ah, the joys of your own personal chef. "She has a personal chef. I want one of those!"

It wasn't long after that delightful encounter that Mitch and his wife moved to the Washington, D.C. area, which was very close to our Annapolis home. I then thought I was set for life with my own wonderful gluten-free personal chef. But then we moved! I don't expect Chef Mitch to follow us here, but he did give me some pointers on finding a personal chef in this region.

One recommendation, was of course, word-of-mouth. Mitch's second recommendation was to find someone associated with the United States Personal Chef Association (USPCA.)

A Personal Chef in Your Kitchen?

Having a personal chef is like having your best friend cooking for you in your own kitchen. This chef knows your special diet. This chef knows your personal likes and dislikes. You can be confident that your meal will be safe and delicious, because this chef is preparing something especially for you.

There are several reasons for having a personal chef. I think the first is obvious: your food is being prepared in your gluten-free zone, your own kitchen. There should be no worries about cross contamination here.

Secondly, in our busy lives, a personal chef brings the convenience of a restaurant meal to you without having to go out to eat.

Thirdly, it eliminates stress. You have no worries about buying ingredients, fretting over a recipe, and getting the meal to the table on time.

And, finally, it is simply wonderful to be pampered on occasion. You can be a guest in your own home. "Miss Janet, your dinner is served." Music to my ears.

The Cost of a Personal Chef

If you're worried about the cost, once you check into the details, I believe you'll find it comparable to eating in a restaurant. In some cases, it may be less. Remember there are no tips to consider, no add-on costs once your settle on a menu and a fixed price, no baby sitters to pay, and no fuel costs for your vehicle. Your price depends on the menu and how formal or exotic or how casual you want to be.

Having a chef prepare family meals once a week, or so, you'll find the cost is not much more than taking the gang out for the evening. There is an additional benefit: your home-cooked meal prepared by your personal chef is adapted to your tastes and requirements, and it is nutritious.

I recommend being up front about the cost. Ask for examples of price ranges for various types of meals, since the price varies widely. A casual family meal consisting of a meat dish with two side dishes costs less than a six course formal dinner. The chefs I interviewed were not at all similar in pricing. Ask first.

Knoxville Area Personal Chefs

The chefs listed in this section have undergone sessions with me in my kitchen concerning in-depth gluten-free requirements. They have each prepared meals for me in my kitchen. I will not give a recommendation here about which personal chef to choose. Choosing a Personal Chef is, well, personal. The recommendation I will make to you, however, is to interview each of your chosen chefs, get to know them, learn how the business works, cost estimates, etc., then make your personal choice. Be sure you are comfortable with the chef's gluten-free knowledge. Let me know what you think.

Raymond Bordelon
www.fruitfulvintagechef.com
865-774-0251
Chef Ray is the chef for Eight Gables Inn in Gatlinburg, a graduate of the Rel Maples Institute for Culinary Arts at Walters State, a member of the United States Personal Chef's Association, and a personal chef. He taught a course in the Guest Chef Series at Walters State and is savvy in cooking gluten free.

Brenda Beaty
bbcooks4u@gmail.com
Brenda, who lives locally, has been cooking for me for several years. She's reliable, trustworthy, and a good cook. She's well versed in the gluten-free diet.

Caterers and Homemade Takeout

This is a new section for alternative good-food sources.

Jill's Healthy Food-To-Go
Jill Hahn is well versed in macrobiotics, vegan, and gluten-free food preparation. She prepares homemade take-out meals. She also offers cooking classes.
You may contact her at
simplyhealthful@yahoo.com

The Casual Gourmet
Tony Britz
4354 Gravelly Hills Rd
Louisville, TN 37777
tonythechef@comcast.net
thecasualgourmet.org
865-980-0160 & 865-591-3952
A quote from Tony: "The Casual Gourmet offers a wide selection of menu ideas that are tailored around your tastes and needs whether they be gluten free, vegetarian, vegan or any other dietary restrictions. From light fare to full course meals and I personalize every dish. Chef Tony."

The Happy Badger Catering Company
Theresa West offers a gluten-free menu using dedicated gluten-free equipment. Her mother has celiac disease and she learned to cook gluten free for her. She fully understands the diet and safe food preparation. Theresa currently has a cafe at 6356 Clinton Hwy, but is considering a move in the near future. Check her website or call for more information.
865-335-7526
facebook page and twitter (@Happybadgerco)
happybadgercateringco.com.

We're cooking gluten-free in East Tennessee! Didn't I tell you this was a special place?

Part 2 Coping with Gluten Intolerance
Excerpts from *Gluten-Free Mainstream America*
Celebrating the Good Food in Gluten Free
Introduction

There are many of us living the good gluten-free life. Who are we? Where are we?

We are everywhere. We are one in 133. We are integrated into every niche, every avenue of society. We are engineers, homemakers, doctors, artisans, factory workers, farmers, scientists, and technicians, male and female from all cultures and age groups. We stand next to you in line at the grocery store. We sit next to you in church. We form the ranks of gluten-free America.

We bond with one another immediately. We network. We share coping techniques and survival tips. We are comrades-in-arms because our lives are on the line. We have celiac disease. We understand one another and the daily challenges we face. If we want to live a healthy life, we must avoid gluten in any form, in any amount ... forever. We have no choice.

For those of us lucky enough to have been diagnosed, it is our job to help one another. It is especially important to help those newly diagnosed to make the transition into the gluten-free life a smooth one. If you are new to celiac disease or non-celiac gluten intolerance, you are not alone. If you need help, reach out. There is someone here to guide you along.

Coping

We each have our unique ways of coping with the new life of gluten free. Immediately upon diagnosis, I declared myself to be a gluten-free zone. My first line of defense against toxic gluten was my kitchen. I knew I was safe in the fortress of my home where I had 100 percent control of everything coming into my kitchen. No toxic foods entered my safety zone. Once I was comfortable within my personal gluten-free zone, and I began to heal, I expanded my zone of safety to include the real world, my neighborhood, my city, my state, and all across America. I began a personal gluten-free awareness campaign to educate everyone and anyone who would take time to listen to me. I developed a restaurant guide for my personal gluten-free awareness campaign, "Miss Janet's Gluten-Free Zone." ® I distributed it to restaurants all across America as I traveled with my husband on business. A few years later, I wrote a book for my community, My Gluten-Free Knoxville, on how to safely live gluten free in our area. As I talked to chefs, restaurant owners, and others sharing my concerns, I experienced compassion and understanding of our gluten-free requirements. My gluten-free zone now includes everywhere I travel throughout America.

What is Gluten, and How Do You Rid It From Your Life?

For recently diagnosed newcomers, this new world can be confusing and somewhat daunting at first. It is here where we, who have experience surviving in a world dominated by gluten-toxic grains, can help the newly initiated down the path to a healthier life style.

Let's begin by telling the rest of the world what we already know. The more people who understand our need for a strict adherence to a gluten-free diet, the safer our food supply will be. Celiac disease is a genetically inherited autoimmune disease. The sub-proteins found in wheat, rye, and barley set off an immune reaction that damages the lining of the intestines, preventing absorption of vital nutrients. That is why celiac disease is also classified as a disease of malnutrition.

A study at the University of Maryland revealed that one American in 133 has celiac disease. It is important for us to remember that this is a hereditary disease, and within our families one in 22 of our immediate relatives could have it as well. Once we have a diagnosis, it's important that our family members get tested for celiac disease. It is a sobering thought to realize that we are seeing only the tip of the iceberg today, because approximately 83 percent of our fellow citizens who have celiac disease don't know it yet.

Symptoms vary, ranging from intestinal pain, bloating, and diarrhea, to hair loss, muscle pain, and weakness. For children a common symptom is a failure to thrive. In the most difficult-to-diagnose cases, there are no symptoms at all until the person develops related diseases, such as osteoporosis or intestinal lymphoma.

Another disorder associated with celiac disease is a skin rash called dermatitis herpetiformis. The chronic red, itchy, blistering rash, often described as celiac disease of the skin, is treated with a gluten-free diet. Although I have been diagnosed with both celiac disease and dermatitis herpetiformis, not everyone with celiac disease has the skin disorder.

Those of us with celiac disease do not have a choice about the foods we eat. We must maintain a strict gluten-free diet for life or risk potential life-threatening consequences down the road.

I'm happy to report that sources for gluten-free foods are becoming more plentiful. Throughout America, I've experienced a high degree of gluten-free awareness. I'm comforted by the sincere efforts to understand our medical requirements, and the willingness to help us succeed.

Helping us also helps the community. It is good for our health. It's good for business. Those of us with celiac disease occupy a large block of consumers. Our disease is twice as common as Crohns' disease, ulcerative colitis, and cystic fibrosis combined. Comparatively, one million Americans have Parkinson's disease. More than two million, possibly as many as three million, Americans have the potential to be affected by celiac disease.

Food manufacturers are beginning to realize our buying potential. When I wrote my first gluten-free guide, *My Gluten-Free Knoxville,* I consulted with Cynthia Kupper, Executive Director of the Gluten Intolerance Group. She explained that an even larger portion of our population suffers from non-celiac gluten intolerance. This group, receiving either negative or inconclusive results with traditional testing for celiac disease, benefits from a gluten-free diet. So when we join our two million Americans with celiac disease together with those who have non-celiac gluten sensitivity, we represent 15 million people. And that's what the food industry recognizes. There is an enormous American market for gluten-free products.

Our ranks are growing daily because of better diagnostic procedures. The demand for gluten-free products will never diminish, rather, the demand will increase as more of us are diagnosed. We aren't the fickle public who will drop the gluten-free lifestyle in a few months, nor are we followers of a trendy fad diet. Once we're on the diet, we will always be gluten-free. It's up to each of us to talk to local grocers and to restaurant owners about our gluten-free requirements. The more people who know about our needs, the safer our food supply will be.

After Diagnosis

What happened when I learned I had a disease that was destroying my intestines and I could never again eat wheat, rye, or barley … and possibly oats? What happened when my doctor told me I have celiac disease and my diet must forever remain gluten free?

My first reaction was relief. I finally knew what I was dealing with. I felt it was news worthy of celebration. My doctor said this disease was something I could control with the proper diet. Food? I could control it with food! I was physically weak, under nourished, and frighteningly frail. The food angle sounded good to me.

My second reaction was confusion. No wheat, no rye, no barley nor any of their derivatives. Oats are not allowed because of the cross-contamination factor: oats are grown and processed close to wheat. Later, I will address the welcome news of developments in the oat world. It's wonderful news for oat lovers.

Wheat was seemingly in everything I enjoyed. Up until the time of my diagnosis, I made my own fresh breads and pastas. The news brought with it the realization that the foods I loved were toxic to me. No more fresh pasta, no rye bread hot out of the oven, no delicious homemade barley soup. What could I possibly eat now? I soon learned that I was not alone in my fears and confusion.

Emotions and Reality

After I got over the fear of the unknown before diagnosis and the relief afterward, other shocks and emotions set in. I felt a deep sense of betrayal. For goodness sake, my own immune system is trying to kill me! Eating is supposed to be health sustaining, not life threatening.

What happened to comfort food? Hot roast beef sandwiches with gravy: gluten filled. The smooth macaroni and cheese casserole: poison. No more bread made with wheat flour, no pizza, no pasta, no oatmeal cereal, no traditional chocolate cake. Even a crumb is toxic. I must avoid gluten in sauces and marinades, barley malt, malt flavoring, broth, bouillon, soy sauce and even self-basting poultry.

Like all others with this disease, I'm fighting hard to put the comfort back into comfort food. I should be able to expect my foods to be safe and I am comforted when I know they are.

Ubiquitous Gluten

Along with the diagnosis of celiac disease comes an education in chemistry and nutrition. We must learn about every aspect of how our food is prepared and every ingredient that goes into it.

It's easy to identify wheat, rye, and barley in their basic forms. We must also avoid the other forms of wheat that are harmful, such as spelt, kamut and triticale. The Food Allergen Labeling and Consumer Protection Act went into effect at the beginning of 2006. Wheat, listed as one of the major allergens, must be identified on the food label. Our lives got easier. By the year 2009, the term "gluten free" was supposed to be defined for food labeling. As of this date in 2013, gluten is still not officially defined. Once it is, food manufactures have the option to list gluten free on food labels if they abide by the definition of the term gluten free.

To someone newly diagnosed, it seems like gluten is lurking even in the most innocent of things, such as a binding and filler ingredient in some medications, an ingredient in multi-vitamins, and even in cosmetics. In a gluten-filled world, there is a lot to learn in order to survive.

Cross Contamination

Cross contamination is a factor to consider in the commercial food processing equation. When I called a company's information line to ask if their chocolates were gluten free, the representative said, "absolutely not." Even though no gluten source was listed in the ingredients on the box, cross contamination in processing had to be considered. She couldn't guarantee that the product was gluten free. I was grateful for her direct response to my inquiry.

Cross contamination can happen in a mill where grains, such as corn and wheat, are processed in close proximity or share the same conveyor belts. It can occur in restaurants at salad bars or in stores with food in open bins. It can occur when a spoon in the croutons bowl is innocently placed into the tomato bin. It can occur when a server slices a piece of bread, then wipes the knife and uses it to slice your naturally gluten-free tomatoes.

Even in our own homes, we must be ever vigilant for cross contamination. In my friend's house, they have a toaster oven for his gluten-free breads, as well as a "family" toaster for wheat breads for everyone else. The family is careful to mark items in the pantry and refrigerator as gluten-free items. In my house, crumbs in the butter dish are not my concern, because my house is a Gluten-Free Zone. Nothing enters that is harmful to me. That's how I got back the comfort in comfort foods. I'm an enthusiastic cook, and no one has ever suffered or complained that the food I prepare is totally gluten free. I know gluten free is good food.

The Healing Process

Once I learned about being gluten sensitive, I joined a support group, talked to doctors, consulted a registered dietitian, researched and read volumes of sometimes confusing and conflicting information. I called consumer 800 numbers for a detailed list of the ingredients in food products.

Cooking is an integral part of my life. I love good food. Because of my love of cooking, this new phase of my life was as easy as making some adjustments, albeit radical at the beginning. My diet prior to diagnosis was balanced with good foods, such as fruits and vegetables, but it was also heavy with toxic grains, bulgur, barley and semolina pasta. Those grains, by the way, went out the door on the first day of my diagnosis.

Good News Foods

Of course, fresh food has always been my main ingredient, and many of my non-grain recipes were already gluten free. I cook with what I call my Good News Foods: foods that are naturally gluten free, including rice, corn, potatoes, vegetables, fruits, and tapioca. I eat fresh non-processed meat, poultry, fish, beans, nuts, milk, eggs, and cheeses. I find much of what I need in the fresh produce section and the fresh meat department of my local markets.

A healthful gluten-free diet consists of many wonderful grains in addition to white rice, brown rice and wild rice. Consider the delicious alternatives of amaranth, buckwheat (bad name: good grain, which contains no wheat), corn, millet, Montina (a native Indian rice grass), oats (uncontaminated, of course), quinoa, sorghum (also called milo), and teff.

Because of the freshness of our foods and the avoidance of processed foods, this diet is a healthful diet for everyone. Cooking with fresh unprocessed whole foods is a natural source of enrichment. The fresh-is-best philosophy works for me. Gluten free is good food.

For those new to the gluten-free lifestyle, I recommend consulting a dietary specialist to ensure you are receiving a proper balance of nutrients from your new diet.

Helping Others

For those who are newly diagnosed, learning about the disease and its treatment can be confusing. There is a lot of misinformation in the public domain. It's much easier sorting it out when there is someone to guide you through the maze. There is help within the celiac disease community. No one needs to feel isolated and alone.

I, therefore, continue to advocate for gluten-free awareness. As an ambassador for seeing the goodness in gluten free, it is, and has been, my goal to integrate gluten-free into Mainstream America. Gluten free should be as common as low-fat, low sodium, and low carbohydrates in our national dialog in restaurants, institutions, and homes across America.

I find comfort in my ability to take control of my illness. There is life after gluten. And it's a good one, at that.

Gluten Free is Good Food

"Let food be thy medicine, and medicine be thy food." Hippocrates

Most foods are naturally gluten free. Eliminating the bad stuff, i.e. wheat, barley, and rye, and any of their derivatives, from our diet is easier than you think.

We know we cannot eat toxic gluten. We can, however, eat everything else! Let's examine all the wonderful things on earth that do not contain gluten. The list of good-for-you food is longer than the list of things that are bad. Here is what is naturally gluten free. Our safe foods include all fresh, non-processed fruits and vegetables and meats. Our safe foods include all types of potatoes, roots and tubers, rice (white, brown, wild), corn, sorghum, tapioca (also known as yucca, cassava, and manioc), buckwheat, amaranth, quinoa, millet, and teff. We can safely eat all fresh, non-processed meats, poultry, fish, beans, legumes, and nuts. Eggs are safe, as well as milk, many cheeses, some yogurts (read your labels), and pure butter. Fresh is Best.

There is no cure for the disease, but it is controlled by strict adherence to a gluten-free diet. Years ago, celiac disease was difficult to diagnose. The medical community and the United States Government have come to the realization that this disease is in epidemic proportions throughout our population. We are now gearing up for better diagnostic tools and better treatment.

Many of us were diagnosed after wasted years of misdiagnoses. Some of the consequences of a late diagnosis include osteoporosis, nerve damage, and intestinal lymphoma. It is a disease to be taken seriously. We must constantly raise awareness that one in 133 Americans are affected. The numbers are growing daily. Remember, more than two million Americans have the potential to have celiac disease. In addition, when we include those with non-celiac gluten intolerance, our ranks expand to 15 million.

I was finally diagnosed with celiac disease after 12 years of health issues directly tied to celiac disease. I am a statistic and good example of a person receiving a late diagnosis. I am not alone. My story is like thousands of others. Today I avoid toxic gluten at all costs.

Being gluten free is not a choice, it is a lifesaving medical necessity. The often repeated quote attributed to Hippocrates, the Father of Medicine, is on target for our gluten-free diet. "Let food be thy medicine, and medicine be thy food." Gluten-free food is our medicine.

Gluten-Free Daily Living Resources

There are many excellent sources for finding accurate and reliable information about celiac disease and gluten-free living. The listings here give you a place to start.

If you have recently been diagnosed, please do what you can to contact your local celiac support group. The good people at your local support group are living the life, walking the walk, talking the talk. They will share coping techniques and helpful tips to help you get started.

It's important that you know you are not alone. We help one another. Information is power. The more information you have, the more powerful you will become in taking control of your new life. It's a good life, this gluten-free living, and we help one another make it so.

Newcomer Pep Talk

If you are recently diagnosed, think of this information as a basic survival course. It is not intended to be an end-all guide. It is your road map for the beginning of your journey. The purpose of this section is simply to help you through your first few days on the diet that will carry you through the rest of your life … a healthy life of good eating.

You can start this very moment to become a Gluten-Free Zone. The information provided here will tide you over while you prepare yourself for the next step of information gathering. You'll see a dietitian who has experience with gluten-free requirements. You'll learn more about your needs through your research and through the advice of others. You'll learn where to find gluten-free foods. You'll learn how to cook with gluten-free products.

Today you can stop the bad stuff from happening. Eliminate the gluten from your life now! Rid your pantry and your refrigerator of anything containing toxins. Look at ingredient listings on boxes of food, cans, bags. Anything that is on the Toxic Foods list (listed below) must be identified. If you plan on making your kitchen a gluten-free zone, put your wheat pastas, your unopened loaves of bread, your canned goods containing things like modified wheat starch into a big grocery bag. Then take the bag to your local church, homeless shelter, or charity drop off center. Give the food to someone who can use it.

If it isn't practical to make your entire kitchen gluten free because of others in your family not wishing to share your diet, then identify all the toxins and keep them from mixing with your foods. Some people have separate shelves in the refrigerator dedicated to their foods. Mark your foods well and keep them from getting cross contaminated. Use separate cooking utensils. Buy yourself a gluten-free designated toaster.

Toxic Foods

Gluten is found in wheat, rye, barley, and grains with names like spelt, kamut, and triticale. Avoid all derivatives of these grains. No pasta, graham, bulgur, or wheat germ. No sauces, gravies, or marinades made with wheat flour thickeners. No breaded coatings, malt, or modified wheat starch.

Note: Common oats are contaminated from being grown and processed near wheat. There are now gluten-free oats that are grown and processed gluten free.

Healthful Foods

White rice, brown rice, wild rice, corn, potatoes, sorghum, tapioca, buckwheat, quinoa, amaranth, teff and millet, and other seeds, such as sunflower, pumpkin, chia, and sesame. We can safely eat plain, non-processed meat, poultry, fish, beans, legumes, nuts, fruits, vegetables, roots and tubers, milk, many cheeses, some yogurts. Vinegar is safe. We can use oils and vinegars on our salads. We can use real butter, and some spreads like Smart Balance Buttery Spread, which is labeled gluten-free.

Gluten-Free Oats

The concern with cross-contamination in oats in the processing and packaging is a valid one. Years ago, when I was first diagnosed, oats were definitely off limits because of cross-contamination. Gluten-free oats are now grown in dedicated gluten-free fields with dedicated equipment and processing. The oats are tested every step of the way in processing and packaging.

Be aware that many doctors believe we should "wade into the waters" carefully when introducing oats back into our diets. Some of us may not be able to tolerate oats as well as others. As you would with any new food being introduced into your diet, first ask your doctor or your dietary specialist, then sample a little, see how you tolerate it. Proceed cautiously until you are sure you can handle it.

National Organizations

Celiac Disease Foundation
Celiac Disease Foundation
20350 Ventura Blvd Ste 240
Woodland Hills CA 91364
Phone: (818) 716-1513
Fax: (818) 267-5577
celiac.org

Gluten-Intolerance Group of North America
31214 124th Ave SE
Auburn, WA 98092-3667
Phone: (253) 833-6655
Fax: (253) 833-6675
gluten.net
Gluten Free Certification Organization: www.gfco.org
Gluten Free Restaurant Awareness Program: www.glutenfreerestaurants.org

National Institutes of Health (NIH)
The National Institutes of Health (NIH) Celiac Disease Awareness Campaign offers a website dedicated to celiac disease awareness: http://celiac.nih.gov

National Digestive Diseases Information Clearinghouse
Bethesda, MD 20892-3570
niddk.nih.gov/health/digest/pubs/celiac/index.htm
(The NDDIC is a service of the National Institute of Diabetes and Digestive and Kidney Diseases (NIDDK), which is part of the National Institutes of Health under the U.S. Department of Health and Human Services.)

National Foundation for Celiac Awareness
You'll find information on education, advocacy, and research. This is a very active group.
celiaccentral.org

Online Shopping

There are several great online sources for gluten-free shopping, including (1) Amazon: amazon.com (I order my Orgran self-rising flour there). Just type in the search window your specific item. Also online, you will find (2) Gluten-Free Trading Company: www.food4celiacs.com or www.gluten-free.tc; and (3) The Gluten-Free Mall: www.celiac.com/glutenfreemall, which are good examples of how easy it is to buy gluten-free foods.

Reference Books & Magazines

There are several excellent reference books and magazines on celiac disease and eating gluten free. Here are a few of my favorites.

Gluten-Free Living

glutenfreeliving.com

This national celiac disease news magazine, backed by an impressive medical advisory board and dietitian advisory board, keeps us informed of research and coping techniques for every-day gluten-free living. Each issue is filled with current and vital information.

Living Without

livingwithout.com

This is an excellent lifestyle guide, heavily focused on celiac disease and food-related allergies. It features delicious recipes and coping techniques and true-life stories of people taking control of their lives in positive ways. Every issue contains powerful information to help us adjust to our required diets.

Gluten-Free Grocery Shopping Guide

ceceliasmarketplace.com

This compact, easy to use shopping guide by Matison & Matison lists more than 25,000 gluten-free products available in mainstream grocery stores, including many over-the-counter pharmacy products.

The Essential Gluten-Free Grocery Guide
triumphdining.com
This guide by TriumphDining helps you find gluten-free products in your grocery store, listing more than 20,000 items.

The Essential Gluten-Free Restaurant Guide, How and Where to Eat Gluten-Free
triumphdining.com
"Featuring celiac-friendly dining across the USA," by Triumph Dining.

Celiac Sprue: A Guide Through the Medicine Cabinet, by Marcia Milazzo
available at Amazon.com, type title in the search window. Since drug manufacturers can change the inactive ingredients on prescription drugs at any time, you need to call the manufacturer each time you get a refill to ensure you have a gluten-free product. This book lists all drug manufacturers in the U.S.

Celiac Disease, A Hidden Epidemic,
"Unmasking one of the most underdiagnosed autoimmune diseases," by Peter H. R. Green, M.D., Director of the Celiac Disease Center at Columbia University, and Rory Jones.

Gluten-Free Diet, A Comprehensive Resource Guide
by Shelley Case, dietitian.

Kids with Celiac disease: A Family Guide to Raising Happy, Healthy, Gluten-Free Children,
by Danna Korn. She also founded R.O.C.K; Raising Our Celiac Kids, a national support group for families of gluten-free children: www.celiackids.com.

Gluten-Free 101, Easy, Basic Dishes Without Wheat
by Carol Fenster, Ph.D.

Online Sources and Apps for Finding Gluten-Free Restaurants

Mobile apps and online sources are cropping up daily. This is just a sampling. Some are free apps, and some costs a few dollars. Go to the websites to download the apps.

Gluten-Free Restaurant Awareness Program: glutenfreerestaurants.org
Gluten-Free Dining Guide: celiacrestaurantguide.com
DineGF: Gluten-free chain restaurant menus and locations: glutenfreetravelsite.com
Locate all things gluten free near you: glutenfreeregistry.com
Yelp. Type in gluten-free restaurants in the search window: yelp.com
Locate allergy friendly restaurants near you: allergyeats.com
Locate chain restaurants, local restaurants, recipes and products: findmeglutenfree.com
Chain restaurants with gluten-free and allergen lists, custom to your needs:
      glutenfreepassport.com: iCanEat OnTheGo Gluten Free & Allergen Free. Another app gives you information on ethnic restaurant ingredients: iEatOut Gluten & Allergen Free

How to "Gluten Free" Everything

Gluten Free Your Kitchen

My kitchen today remains a gluten-free zone. It became my haven of gluten free the minute I came home from being diagnosed with celiac disease in the year 2000. The day I was diagnosed I methodically searched my refrigerator and my pantry, removing every gluten-containing item. I placed the unopened items in grocery bags and took them downtown to a shelter for women. I threw out anything that was opened.

What I discovered on that day was a large portion of food in the kitchen pantry contained gluten. Cans of tomato soup, chicken noodle soup, cream of chicken soup, all pastas and flours, cake mixes, mayonnaise, and even chicken and beef stocks contained derivatives of toxic gluten. In contrast to the processed foods in my pantry that were now off limits to me, I found a bounty of naturally gluten-free fresh foods in the refrigerator and in the fruit basket on the kitchen counter. I immediately named them my *good-news foods*: fresh fruits and vegetables; white and brown rice; unprocessed chicken, beef, and pork; walnuts, almonds, and sunflower seeds; eggs, cheese, and milk. There are more good-news foods that I have discovered since my early days of gluten free, such as quinoa, millet, buckwheat, chia seeds, sorghum, and flours, such as tapioca flour, almond flour, and coconut flour.

Food had once been the source of my ills. Now food became the foundation of my plan to regain my health and take control of my life once again. From that day forth, my home became a gluten-free zone, a welcome retreat from the very scary real world of a gluten-dominated society. Ridding my home of the gluten that was killing me (I was gravely ill at the time of my diagnosis) gave me the sense of complete control over my destiny. Inside my kitchen there was no threat of cross contact/cross contamination. Inside my kitchen I found only wholesome, safe food. I found my medicine for recovery.

Today we have federal labeling laws. If a food product contains wheat in any form, it must be written on the label saying so. You will see words and phrases, such as,

- Contains wheat.
- Made in a facility that also processes wheat.
- This product is made on machinery where wheat products are processed.

The allergen labeling law is one giant step for our gluten-intolerant community. As of this writing, the law for labeling gluten is still pending. Hopefully in the near future, if a product contains any form of gluten, it must be designated on the label.

My advice for checking the foods in your kitchen for safety is to **read every label** carefully. The chore is easier now because of the allergen labeling laws. However, until we have the long-awaited law that requires all gluten sources to be listed, we must remain vigilant. Wheat, rye, and barely are easy to spot when spelled out like that. But remember malt is made from barley. Innocent things like chocolate malted balls are off limits to us. Rye bread, barley soup, malt and hops in beer are also off limits. We must also avoid the other forms of wheat that are harmful, such as spelt, kamut and triticale.

Making your kitchen a gluten-free zone is easy if everyone in the household is gluten free. However, there are households living in both worlds with gluten and non gluten. If that is your case, cross contamination is a constant issue that must be addressed by everyone in the household. You must keep your gluten-free foods safe from cross contact/cross contamination. Perhaps you will designate a separate shelf in the refrigerator as gluten free. You will have a separate gluten-free toaster and/or toaster oven. You will be careful to prevent crumbs in the butter dish. And you will take measurers to never place a wheat-contaminated knife in the gluten-free peanut butter jar.

If you are recently diagnosed, I recommend that you become an avid label reader. I recommend you study hard to recognize all sources of gluten. And I recommend that you become your own advocate for gluten-free awareness to keep yourself safe at all times.

Gluten Free Your Recipes

The recipes I produce contain naturally gluten-free ingredients. However, when I list an ingredient that is processed, such as mayonnaise, **it is up to you to read the label** or **call the manufacturer** to make sure the product you are using is gluten free. The same goes for the breads and flours listed within the recipes. Check your labels on anything that is processed, such as prepared flour mixes to ensure they are gluten free. If my recipe calls for flour, think gluten-free flour. If it calls for bread crumbs, think gluten-free bread crumbs. **Read the labels** on pre-made items every time you purchase them. I cook gluten free and I am able to use every recipe in any cookbook by using gluten-free ingredients. **Everything can be converted to gluten free just by using your "noodle!"**

Author Profile

Janet McKenzie Prince is a niche-market independent publisher dealing with varied subjects, such as wildlife rescue, pet rescue and adoption, celiac disease, food and health.

Through her Gluten-Free Awareness Campaign, Miss Janet's Gluten-Free Zone™, she offers advice and educational materials to restaurant owners and chefs about gluten-free cooking. She promotes celiac disease awareness within the medical community. And she helps those recently diagnosed to ease into their new gluten-free lifestyle through her guides, *My Gluten-Free Knoxville* and *Gluten-Free Mainstream America*.

In her book, *New Cooks in America*, Prince invites America back into the kitchen where good stuff happens; where food cures your ills, not causes your ills; and where cooking is fun and easy. *New Cooks in America* was launched to entice Americans, young and old alike, to return to the kitchen for a healthier America.

Prince remains active in supporting pet rescue and pet adoption. Her books, *Duff at First Sight* and *Watching Heather Bloom* were used to raise awareness for the plight of homeless pets. All of her rescue dogs are living proof that older dogs make wonderful pets, as well as demonstrate that you *can* teach old dogs new tricks. She and her husband currently share quarters with two rescued Westies and one little brown stray, who, she says, "arrived one cold December day, unpacked her bags, and stayed."

Through her publication studio, Prince published two books on wildlife rescue written by her mother, Marjorie McKenzie Davis, founder of Wildlife Fawn Rescue in Kenwood, California. She published *Leap to Freedom* in 1998, and *Setting the Fawn Free* in 2010.

As a career journalist, Prince has served as a travel correspondent and photographer in the United States as well as in Mexico, and a newspaper columnist and feature writer in Pennsylvania. With concentrations in the fields of print journalism, publication design and production, she holds a bachelor's degree from the University of Maryland and a master's degree from Yale Gordon College at the University of Baltimore.

She lives with her husband, dogs, cats, and abundant wildlife on their property outside of Knoxville in East Tennessee.

Books by the Author
Bienvenido a Mexico! 1977, Gilbert Commonwealth
Day Trips Out of Reading, 1982, Reading Eagle Company
Pennsylvania Highlights, 1984, Reading Eagle Company
How to Discover Berks County, 1985, Reading Eagle Company
New Cooks on the Block, 1992, Cottage of Arts in Annapolis
New Cooks II, 1997, Cottage of Arts in Annapolis
Duff at First Sight, 1999, Burley Creek Studio
Watching Heather Bloom, 1999, Burley Creek Studio
My Gluten-Free Knoxville, first edition 2008, Revised 2013, White Dog Studio
New Cooks in America, 2012, White Dog Studio
Miss Janet's American Breadbasket, 2013, White Dog Studio
Gluten-Free Mainstream America, 2013, White Dog Studio

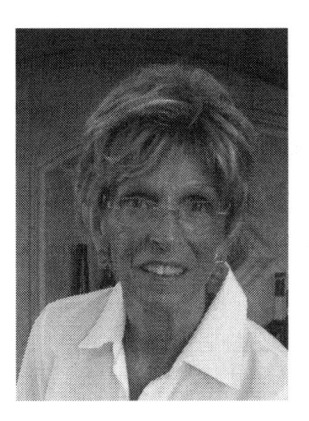

www.missjanetsglutenfreeamerica.com

Made in the USA
Charleston, SC
03 August 2013